YOUR KNOWLEDGE HAS VALUE

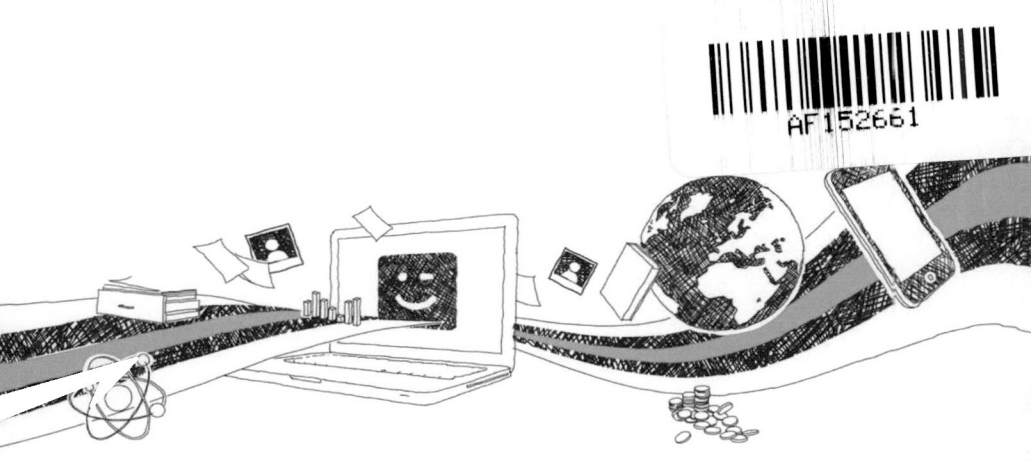
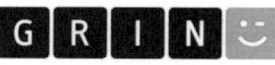

Peter Okeke

The Rhesus Negative Pregnant Mothers and Haemolytic Disease of Newborn (HDN) among Neonatals born in Central Hospital Porto Novo

GRIN Publishing

Bibliographic information published by the German National Library:

The German National Library lists this publication in the National Bibliography; detailed bibliographic data are available on the Internet at http://dnb.dnb.de .

Imprint:

Copyright © 2010 GRIN Verlag GmbH
Print and binding: Books on Demand GmbH, Norderstedt Germany
ISBN: 978-3-640-79282-5

This book at GRIN:

http://www.grin.com/en/e-book/163579/the-rhesus-negative-pregnant-mothers-and-haemolytic-disease-of-newborn

GRIN - Your knowledge has value

Since its foundation in 1998, GRIN has specialized in publishing academic texts by students, college teachers and other academics as e-book and printed book. The website www.grin.com is an ideal platform for presenting term papers, final papers, scientific essays, dissertations and specialist books.

Visit us on the internet:

http://www.grin.com/

http://www.facebook.com/grincom

http://www.twitter.com/grin_com

THE RHESUS NEGATIVE PREGNANT MOTHERS AND HAEMOLYTIC DISEASE OF NEWBORN (HDN) AMONG NEONATALS BORN IN CENTRAL HOSPITAL PORTO NOVO.

BY
OKEKE PETER UBAH
2010

ABSTRACT

A total of 27 blood specimen of neonates born at the maternity section of central Hospital Porto Novo by the Rhesus Negative mothers were studied for a period of 12 months. The specimen collection were done within 72 hours of birth, mothers pregnant for the first time without a past history of abortion or transfusion were rejected for the study. Ten (10) blood specimens of the neonates were Rhesus blood group negative and were eliminated from the work whereas the remaining seventeen (17) were recorded Rhesus blood group positive.

The results of the 17 specimen of neonates all recorded in mean values showed Hb 17. 23g/dl, Hct 51.56L/L, the mean cell volume was 102.18 FL, mean cell hemoglobin concentration was 33.41% and mean cell hemoglobin recorded 34.12 pg. The red cell count and white cell count were $5.04 \times 10^{12/L}$ and 16.06×10^{9}/L respectively. The platelet count was 316.53 and red cell distribution width of 17.76% was recorded. The differential leucocytes counts were; Neutrophils 65.35%, Lymphocytes 25.71% and MXD (comprises of monocytes, eosinophils and basophils) recorded 13.48%.

The mean results of Bilirubin direct and Bilirubin total were 0.76mg/dl and 4.29mg/dl. The Direct Coombs test (DCT) was positive in one specimen of neonates and this specimen showed Hb value of 13.6g/dl and a total Bilirubin of 27.5mg/dl. All the neonates were of full term with birth weight of 2.5 to 3.5 kg. This work serves as an epidemiological vigilance for haemolytic diseases of the newborn in the Porto Novo province.

The incidence of hemolytic Disease of newborn in Porto Novo district was recorded to be 5.8% considering from this work where only a case gave positive Direct Coombs. Although, this work suffers from scarcity of pregnant mothers of Rhesus blood group negative and affects the research because the specimen collected were small for the time period of the work. The Porto Novo experience also showed that good control system is at work by the medical team and technical staff concerned with the testing of all prospective mothers. Another positive aspect is that anti-D is freely and timely available for mothers of D-positive infants and with persistent effort in this regard, the incidence should continue very low or until there is no more case of hemolytic disease of the newborn.

Introduction

The term hemolytic disease of the newborn (HDN) is used to describe an immune hemolytic anemia which causes an infant to be born anemic and jaundiced.
However, Rhesus HDN is usually caused by immune anti-D and less commonly by other Rhesus antibodies. It occurs when a RH negative woman with circulating IgG anti-D antibody (formed from a previous Rhesus incompatible pregnancy) becomes pregnant with a RH positive infant and IgG anti-D passes into the fetal circulation, destroying fetal cells. The infant can be born severely anemic and jaundiced. The severity of the disease increases with each RH positive pregnancy. Infants with Rhesus HDN are usually more severely affected than that caused by other antibodies.

Megan Rowley &Clare Milkins (2006) stated that since immunoglobulin G (igG) is the only immunoglobulin that crosses the placenta, only red cells of antibodies of this class are a potential cause of HDN.

In the RH system, antibodies are formed much more readily against the D-antigen than against any other antigens, so over 99% of infants with RH hemolytic disease will be the RH (D) positive offspring of RH (D) negative mothers.

Professor A.V. Hoff brand (1986) reported the incidence of infants affected with RH HDN in the United Kingdom to be about 0.5-0.75% of all births, although the figures are now falling with the success of routine prophylaxis with anti-D. Of the affected infants,10-20% are born dead or dying if no intrauterine treatment is given and over half of the affected infants need treatment, Often urgently, during the neonatal period. Obviously, it is important to detect the antibodies in the mothers' serum during the antenatal period.

Dr.Sheila Worlledge reported that antibodies due to RH (D) cannot normally be detected during the first pregnancy unless the mother has had previous transfusions and or abortions.

Dr.Nevanlinna has shown that even after five or more pregnancies, the incidence of antibody formation in D- negative women is only about 10.2%.This discrepancy has three basic explanations:
Firstly, not all D-negative women have D-positive children. It can be calculated that in the United Kingdom, about 10% of mating will result in a mother who is D-negative carrying a D-positive fetus and that only 47% of D-negative pregnant for the second time will be carrying a second D-positive child.
Secondly, not all pregnancies are ABO compatible and there is good evidence that ABO-incompatibility protects against RH antibody formation.

Professor Murray (1965) calculated that A-incompatibility gave 90% protection and B-incompatibility affords 55% protection against RH immunization.
The first ABO compatible D-incompatible infant seems to result in the primary immunization of about 17% of RH negative women: In about half of these women, the antibodies appear within six months of delivery; the other half, the antibodies will be detectable by the end of the second pregnancy.

Dr.Worlledge (1983) also stated that abortion produces immunization in up to 4% of D-negative women and the incidence seems to be greater if the abortion occurs in the second trimester than in the first.

ANTENATAL ASSESSMENT OF THE MOTHER´S BLOOD.

All mothers should have their ABO and RH (D) groups determined as soon as possible after pregnancy has been diagnosed. Moreover, their sera should be tested for antibodies outside the ABO blood group system, regardless of their blood group. One suitable way is to test them at 37^{oc} with pooled enzyme treated red cells which have been taken from not more than three donors who between them carry all the common blood group antigens except A and B.
If properly done, this test is very sensitive method for detecting RH antibodies.

However, since other antibodies may have equal importance and since some of the antigens against which the react are destroyed by enzyme treatment, at least selected sera should also be tested with the same untreated red cells by the indirect antiglobulin test (IAT). It is customary for this selection to include the sera from all RH negative mothers and all mothers who give a history of past transfusion or unexplained stillborn, jaundiced or anemic infants.

If these investigations are negative, the sera of RH(D) positive mothers need not be reexamined routinely during pregnancy provided the mothers give no history of past transfusions or infants that might have been affected with hemolytic disease of the newborn. RH (D) negative mothers in their first pregnancy are unlikely to form detectable antibodies until after delivery and their sera probably need to be retested only at 30-40 weeks of pregnancy. RH (D) negative mothers in their second or subsequent pregnancy should be tested more frequently and earlier in pregnancy, Suggested times for these investigations are at 20 weeks and two or three times during the third trimester of pregnancy. All RHD negative mothers who seem to be un- immunized during pregnancy should have their sera retested at delivery if prophylactic anti-D is to be given. The sera of all mothers who give a history of past transfusions or stillborn, jaundiced or anemic infants should also be retested frequently during pregnancy. In these situations, the mother's serum should be tested with the husband´s red cells if no antibodies are found with the pooled cells.

If the preliminary investigations are positive or if positive results are found in any of the subsequent tests, further tests will depend on the specificity of the antibodies. Some antibodies such as anti-Lewis and anti-p1 are almost always Igm and as such will not lead to HDN.

However, their presence should be recorded because they may make subsequent compatibility tests more difficult but the sera need not be titrated. Although haemolytic disease of newborn resulting from anti-D is the most severe form of the disease anti-c can give rise to significant haemolysis inutero sufficient to cause intra uterine death and to warrant investigation in pregnancy. Other antibodies such as RH antibodies, anti-kell, anti-Duffy, anti-E, anti-ce, and anti-Kidd are often IgG and uncommonly give rise to fetal haemolysis of sufficient severity to merit antenatal intervention and if they react by the indirect antiglobulin test, the sera should be titrated against suitable red cells. All pregnant mothers whether D positive or D negative should be screened for red cell antibodies. Further testing depends on the specificity of any antibodies detected, whether they are capable of causing haemolytic disease of the newborn. Antibody titres are now applied, along with the previous history, to decide whether or not to examine the amniotic fluid.

At a reputable Hammersmith Hospital London, a titre of 16 or more as estimated by the indirect antiglobulin method is an indication for amniocentesis and once this titre is reached, further titre need not be done. Previously, the titre was the only guide to the severity of the hemolytic process in the infant. At Hammersmith Hospital London, if the antiglobulin titre of the RH antibodies was 32 or less at 34-36 weeks of gestation, the infant if affected, was unlikely to have serious disease. However, if the titre was 256 or over at 34-36 weeks of pregnancy, the prognosis was bad and one third of the affected infants were born dead.

Dr.Rosenfield (1969) reported that amounts of RH antibody below 0.05 microgram per millitre in the maternal serum at 27-34 weeks of gestation indicate an RH negative or unaffected RH positive infant, while amounts above 0.45 microgram per millitre indicate a very severely affected infant.
Rosenfield (1969) also suggests that 0.2 microgram per millitre of Rh antibody should be the level at or above which amniocentesis should be done.

PARTNER TESTING
The paternal blood group phenotype should be determined in all cases in which the mother has a clinically significant red cell alloantibody. If the paternal red cells lack the corresponding antigen, the baby is not at risk. However, caution is advised because the assumed parent may not be the biological father of the fetus. It is useful to predict whether the partner of a woman who is D negative and who has anti D is homozygous or heterozygous for the D antigen. This helps to forecast the chances of having children affected by anti-D haemolytic disease of the newborn(HDN).

No Antisera against the, d, antigen are available because the d allele does not exist. Because of the lack of anti-d serum, the zygosity of the D antigen is usually predicted from the results of tests with anti-c, anti-C, anti-e and anti-E and from the likelihood of the homozygous or heterozygous association with these antigens. Because the genetic basis for the common D types is now known, DNA typing provides a better alternative for predicting the potential for haemolytic disease of the newborn.

Testing Fetal Deoxyribonucleic acid (DNA) in the maternal circulation.

It is now possible to detect fetal DNA in maternal circulation and using DNA amplification techniques to obtain D and K types on these cells. This has proved to be accurate at predicting the D type and in the United Kingdom it is now offered as a clinical service at the beginning of the second trimester. This may replace more invasive tests and supplement partner typing. It can be especially helpful if the partner is absent or unknown.

ANTENATAL ASSESSMENT OF THE SEVERITY OF HDN

There has been considerable change in antenatal assessment of the severity of HDN in recent years. Many new non-invasive tests have been developed to assess the degree of fetal anaemia and if necessary, to proceed to intrauterine transfusion in severely affected cases.

ANTIBODY TITRATIONS DURING PREGNANCY

In some laboratories, tube techniques have been replaced by column agglutination technology or solid phase microplates.The role of the lab serologist is to carry out serial antibody measurements to determine changes in the titre or concentration of the antibody. It is recommended that the technique chosen for the titration should be validated against the

National institute for biological standards and control anti-D standard. Hence, labs should ensure that titres obtained with the anti-D standard are always within one doubling dilution when it is used as an internal control. In addition, antibody titrations performed in pregnancy should always be performed in parallel with the previous sample. Increases in titres of more than one doubling dilution should always be monitored in conjunction with obstetrician.

ANTIBODY QUANTITATION

Individual labs should work closely with reference labs and obstetricians. Automated quantification is considered to be a more accurate predictor of when to proceed to more active investigation of the fetus but is usually only available for anti-D and sometimes anti-c. Other investigative methods available for predicting fetal risk include cellular assays such as the monocytes monolayer assay and the antibody- dependent cytotoxicity assay as models of in vivo haemolysis in the fetus.

METHOD OF ASSESSMENT OF FETAL ANAEMIA

In a mother with increasing antibody levels and a fetus suspected or known to carry the red cell antigen against which the antibody is directed, an assessment of the severity of haemolysis is required. Traditionally, this was done using amniocentesis to measure the optical density of the amniotic fluid (lilley´s lines) using spectrophotometry. This is an indirect measurement, whereas direct fetal blood sampling by ultrasound guided cordocentesis provides not only direct diagnostic information but also a new approach to fetal therapy by direct fetal intravascular transfusion. However, both of these procedures carry the risk of miscarriage and further fetomaternal haemorrhage. More recently, specialist units have been able to offer noninvasive tests to determine fetal anaemia using middle cerebral artery a method of Doppler(2002)
The incidence and severity of anti-D haemolytic disease of the newborn is declining and the increasingly specialized management of severely affected pregnancies has meant that these women are now being referred to specialist centre dealing with this condition early in pregnancy.

Amniocentesis

A more reliable indicator of fetal jeopardy than maternal anti-D levels is measurement of amniotic fluid bilirubin when the absorbance of normal amniotic fluid is estimated at different wavelengths over the range of 350 nm to 700nm and the curve is plotted on semi-logarithmic graph paper, a smooth progression in absorbance from the lowest figure at 700 nm to the highest at 350 nm is obtained, fluid from a pregnant woman severely affected by HDN causes a bulge in the curve with a peak at 450 nm. The magnitude of the increase absorption at 450 nm is related to the likely severity of haemolysis in the fetus.
Lilely (1961) suggested that the results with amniotic fluid from affected fetuses could be divided into three groups on the basis of the increased absorbance at 450 nm
   1. When there is only slight or no increase in absorbance the infant is not at risk
   2. When the increase is moderate the infant is only at low risk
   3. When the increase is marked the infant is usually seriously affected and at great risk of intra uterine death
It is these babies that could require an intra uterine transfusion if they are to survive. If the fetus is found to be in the minimal risk group, amniocentesis should be repeated in two weeks. Once risk fetus is identified therapeutic intervention is required.

World Health Organization Special Advice on Rhesus Sensitization

A scientific group of the world health organization has recommended that IgG anti-D should be given to all D-negative mothers who have not already been immunized to the D-antigen and who give birth to a D-positive infant. They also recommend that all D-negative women who have abortions should be similarly treated unless the abortion can be proved to be D-negative. The treatment should be as soon as possible after delivery and or abortion with 72 hours.

For women having an abortion at under 12 weeks pregnancy, a dose of 50 microgram anti-D is recommended, for later abortions the usually dose is recommended.

More over, all D-negative women who have any incidents in pregnancy that may lead to appreciable hemorrhage for example, external version, amniocentesis and Ante-Partum Hemorrhage (APH) should be given the recommended dose of anti-D at once. The dose recommended by WHO is 200-300 microgram which is introduced by intramuscular injection.

These are rather sweeping recommendations and supplies may be short in some countries, so the dose of anti-D should be 100 microgram and this will protect very nearly the same number of patients.

Source of anti-D

The anti-D required for prophylaxis is usually obtained from volunteer men and women unable to bear children preferably already immunized. They are deliberately restimulated with D-positive red cells and are bled by plasmapheresis.

MATERIALS AND METHOD

A total of twenty – seven blood specimen were collected and grouped and further test were carried out on seventeen of them.

Automated cell counting instrument – SYSMEX KX-21-N
1. Graduated pipettes
Pasteur pipettes
2. Automatic pipettes
3. Dipotassium ethylenediamine tetra –acetic acid tubes
4. Tube stand and conical tubes
5. Semi –automatic photometer- Humalyser 3000
6. Laminas and cover slips
7. Anti-A, Anti-B, Anti-A/B, Anti-D, anti-sera for blood grouping
8. Antihuman globulin sera
9. Khan tubes
10. Chronometer
11. Bilirubin reagent
12. Physiological saline
13. Centrifuge digital – Labofuge
14. Microscope
15. Blood collection sets
16. Hand gloves
17. Human control sera N and P.

METHOD

Since the hematological profiles are done automatically, the method of bilirubin determination and direct coombs test are stated below:

Bilirubin Determination
Composition:
1.100ml reagent Bilirubin total-white cap.
2. 9ml reagent T-nitrite-white cap.
3.100ml reagent Bilirubin Direct – blue cap.
4. 9ml reagent D-nitrite –blue cap.

BILIRUBIN TOTAL
Pipette as Follows:

TUBES	BLANK	STANDARD OR SAMPLE
REAGENT 1	1000 MICROLITRE	SAME AS BLANK
REAGENT 2	----	A DROP
SAMPLE	100 MICROLITRE	SAME AS BLANK

Treat controls pathological (P) and controls normal (N) as tests were treated. Mix carefully and allow at room temperature for 10 to 30 minutes and read in the humalyser 3000 Colorimeter test reference number 4.Record results.

BILIRUBIN DIRECT
Pipette as Follows:

TUBES	BLANK	STANDARD OR SAMPLE
REAGENT 1	1000 MICROLITRE	SAME AS BLANK
REAGENT 2.	......	A DROP
SAMPLE	100MICROLITRE	SAME AS BLANK

Treat controls (P) and (N) sera same as sample. Mix carefully allows for exactly 5 minutes at room temperature and read in the colorimeter test reference number 4.Record results.

DIRECT COOMBS TEST

- ➤ Wash a 2-5% cell suspension of the infant´s red cells four times in physiological saline.
- ➤ Decant the final supernatant fluid.
- ➤ Resuspend the packed cells.
- ➤ Add two volumes of AHG reagent into a tube containing two volumes of 2-5% cell suspension and mix.
- ➤ Centrifuge at 1500 rpm for 1 minute.
- ➤ Tilting the tube back and front, examine for agglutination macro and microscopically.
- ➤ Treat control IgG sensitized cells same as test
- ➤ A positive direct coombs test indicates antibody coating of the infant´s red cells.

RESULTS

A total of seventeen blood specimens of neonates born by the Rhesus negative mothers were tested for complete blood count (CBC), Bilirubin determination and Direct Coombs test (DCT) and the results were presented as follows:

Table 1- presents the results of complete blood count ...Hematological test.

TEST	Rbc $\times 10^{9/L}$	Hb g/dl	Hct L/L	Wbc $\times 10^{9/L}$	MCV FL	MCH Pg	MCHC g/dl	PLT $\times 10^{9/L}$	Lymph %	MXD %	Neut %	RDW %
TOTAL	85.74	293.0	876.40	273.0	1,737	580.0	568.0	5,381	437.1	229.1	1,111	302.0
MEAN	5.04	17.23	51.56	16.06	102.18	34.12	33.41	316.53	25.71	13.48	65.35	17.76

Table 2-Presents the results of Bilirubin Determination (Bilirubin Direct & Bilirubin Total)

TEST	BD mg/dl	BT mg/dl
TOTAL	13.0	73.0
MEAN	0.76	4.29

Table 3-Presents the results of Direct Coombs Test (DCT)

TEST	DCT
POSITIVE	1
NEGATIVE	16
TOTAL	17

DISCUSSION

They results of the seventeen (17) neonates tested in this research showed the Hb concentration of 17.23g/dl, Haematocrit 51.56L/L, mean cell volume 102.2FL, mean cell haemoglobin 34.12 Pg, mean cell haemoglobin concentration 33.41% and red cell distribution width of 17.8%. The platelet count recorded 316.53 and the white cell count of 16.06×10^9L and the red cell count of $5.04 \times 10^{12/L}$ were both recorded. The leukocytes differential count showed; Neutrophils 65.35%, lymphocytes 25.71%, MXD (comprises of Monocytes, Eosinophils, and Basophils) recorded 13.48%. All these values above were recorded as mean values.

However, the bilirubin direct was 0.76mg/dl and bilirubin total was 4.29mg/dl mean values respectively. Newborns at the Porto Novo district are within 0.5 to 3.0mg/dl reference range of cord blood bilirubin level. The specimen of a neonate showed Direct Coombs test (DCT) positive with a total bilirubin level of 27.5mg/dl and this must have contributed to a little increase in mean total bilirubin, for this reason this work recorded 5.8% incidence of Rhesus haemolytic disease of newborn.

The hyperbilirubinaemia could cause neonatal jaundice as a result of Haemolytic Disease of newborn usually from Rhesus blood group incompatibility and delay formation of the enzymatic conjugating capacity of the liver, principally bilirubin-UDP glucuronosyltransferase. When there is haemolysis, the unconjugated bilirubin may exceed 30mg/dl and above this value, the deposition of the lipid- soluble bilirubin in the basal ganglia is likely and this could lead to the dangerous kernicterus and the level of 30mg/dl is taken as the indication for exchange transfusion. Although kernicterus could occur at a lower level of bilirubin due to the displacement of bilirubin from albumin by certain drugs. Phototherapy is generally recommended to lower bilirubin levels in neonates when this happen. It is worthy to note that all the neonates tested recorded a normal birth weight of 2.5 to 3.5 kg and all the values obtained from complete blood count are within the reference range for neonates.

Although antibodies to almost all known antigens have been reported as causing haemolytic disease of the newborn but by far the commonest clinically important antibody provided by pregnancy is anti-D made by D-negative women. Antibodies cannot normally be detected during the first pregnancy unless the mother has had previous transfusion or abortion and for this reason, only D-negative women that were in the second pregnancy upwards were acceptable in this research. This work was affected because low incidence of D-negative women in population of Porto Novo and also the rejection of first pregnant women, all these contributed to small specimen recorded during this work.

The incidence of haemolytic disease of newborn in Porto Novo was 5.8% with only a positive Direct Coombs test and this neonate that was DCT positive, was normal without any clinical features of haemolytic disease of newborn. Why was this possible? Yes, there could be various reasons but the principal issues could be that, not all pregnancies are ABO compatible and there is good evidence that ABO incompatibility protects against Rhesus antibody formation and it could be that no fetal red cells or too little cells could have gotten into the circulation of the mother and this proves insufficient to stimulate antibody formation , although showed a positive reaction to Direct Coombs test but the neonate was normal in appearance or it could be that the antibodies to anti –D persisted even after anti-D injection as is always the case with IgG. Here in Porto Novo, Cape Verde all D- negative mothers pass through vigorous control system. Those mothers with indirect Coombs positive ante natal, receives 200 to 300µg of immunoglobulin anti-D intramuscularly at 28 and 34 weeks of pregnancy and an additional dose after delivery if the infant proves to be D-positive. We should recall that not all D-negative women have D-positive infants.

Finally, we could comfortably state that the incidence of haemolytic disease of newborn in Porto Novo Hospital is drastically low thanks to the good medical and technical watch out in identifying and medically following up of all D-negative mothers and thanks to the Ministry of Health Cape Verde for good political engagement in providing anti-D freely and timely available at affordable rate to the needy.

CONCLUSION

The results of 5.8% from this study was good but all medical, nursing and technical staff should continue to be on the watch for haemolytic disease of newborn. Correct identification of women in early pregnancy who are D-negative offers the chance to give intramuscular anti-D immunoglobulin to prevent sensitization to the D-antigen at times during the pregnancy when significant fetomaternal haemorrhage is likely to occur. Accuracy in D grouping is particularly important because women who are D-negative erroneously grouped as D positive stands risk of not receiving prophylactic anti-D or being transfused with D positive cells. This could lead to a sensitization to D antigen and could result in severe haemolytic disease of newborn as a result of development of anti-D in subsequent pregnancies.

Anti-D should be given routinely as soon as possible after delivery but always within 72 hours of birth to women who are D negative that give birth to D positive infants. It should also be given after an abort and during termination of pregnancy, chorionic villus sampling and amniocentesis and following any abdominal trauma. It should once again be given for episodes of vaginal bleeding where the pregnancy remains viable.

At delivery and for sensitizing events after 20 weeks of gestation, it is necessary to quantitate the fetomaternal haemorrhage using an acid elution or flow cytometry method so that extra anti-D can be given if the standard dose in use does not cover the estimated bleed. The typing of fetal DNA in the maternal circulation may be used in the near future to select women with fetuses that are D positive that would benefit from this additional prophylaxis of 28 and 34 weeks or a single larger dose at 28 weeks in addition to the postnatal dose, but at the moment, it is not universally offered. It is therefore important to take the 28 weeks sample for blood group and antibody screen before the administration of the anti-D injection.

The Coombs testing of all suspected cases will continue and the medical team should continue to look out for its symptoms and always request the testing as soon as possible, although the case of Porto Novo is different because here in Porto Novo, pregnant mothers are strenuously observed for this.

REFERENCES

1. Bowman.J.M.(1975)
Rh erythroblast sis fetalis, Seminars in Hematology 12:189

2. Clarke C.A. (1975)
Rhesus hemolytic disease selected papers and extracts, Lancaster; medical &technical publishing.

3. Hoffbrand .A.V: and Pettit.J.E (1993)
Essential hematology 3rd ed. *oxford Blackwell scientific*

4. *Liley.A.W :(1961)*
Liquor amnii analysis in management of pregnancy complicated by Rhesus sensitization American Journal of obstetrics and gynecology 82; 1359.

5. Lehman.C.A.(1998)Saunders manual of clinical laboratory sciences,W.B.saunders pg.512

6. Murray.S., Knox &Walker.(1965)
Hemolytic disease and the Rhesus genotypes vox sanguinis (Basel), 10; 257

7. Rosenfield, R.E.(1969)
The current status of some human blood group problems, textbook of immunopathology vol.11

8. Robertson.J.G. (1971)
Diagnosis and management of Rh-immunized patients, J.T: clinical obstetrics and gynecology, 14:494

9. Robinson.E.A. And Tovey .L.A. (1980)
Intensive plasma exchange in the management of severe Rh disease, British Journal of Haematology, 45:621.

10. Tomilinson.J., James S, & wagstaff.w. (1981)
A survey of maternal anti-D levels related to hemolytic disease of the newborn, British Journal of Haematology, 49; 130.

11. Megan Rowley et al (2006)
Antenatal serology and HDN in practical hematology 10th edn by S M Lewis pg540-544.